Nurstoons

The Art of Nursing 2

Carl Elbing
Copyright © 2012 Carl Elbing

All rights reserved.

ISBN: 1478241713
ISBN-13: 978-1478241713

DEDICATED TO **MARK ELBING** AND **SHAWN LAFFERTY**

My cousin Shawn and brother Mark were both tremendous influences in my life. I would never have become who I am without them. I drew pictures with Shawn my entire life; we would spend entire days and evenings drawing monsters, dragons, or other strange creatures that crept into our imaginations. We had a great deal of imaginary adventures and could always rely on our "everything box" that contained... well... *everything* an adventurer could possibly need to get out of trouble when touring the universe and encountering aliens. All three of us spent countless evenings philosophizing about cosmology, religion, the meaning of life... well, pretty much everything. As Mark, Shawn, and I grew older, Mark and Shawn decided to learn how to design webpages and work with graphics (back when the Internet was new). Mark started an online business and taught me the basics of computer graphics and web design. Mark and Shawn worked on a website in which they were going to modify photographs with art programs for people. Mark wanted to put up a website containing my cartoons as a first attempt at a web design; we called it "The Official Nurstoon Homepage". He named his website design business *Fineline Productions*. The website turned out pretty well (at least, we thought so) and contained e-cards, a message board, et cetera... all of which were cutting edge at the time. The website did surprisingly well thanks to all of you out there with a sense of humor as twisted as ours. We put up some cartoons that I had drawn for *The Journal of Nursing Jocularity* and started drawing new cartoons. Mark enjoyed coloring the cartoons, which I hated doing, so this worked out well.

Tragically, Shawn was killed in a car accident; I had the great honor of being the last person to speak with him. As per tradition, we spent our last evening together philosophizing on the usual subjects. Shortly after this, Mark died from an intracranial bleed as a result of his life-long struggle with diabetes. They were two of the most talented people I had known and I was very lucky to have been able to spend so much time with them. There is so much I could say and so much I could write. This paragraph does little justice to the depth of Shawn or Mark or their importance to me. I will miss both of them forever. I can say with great certainty that I would never have become who I am without them.

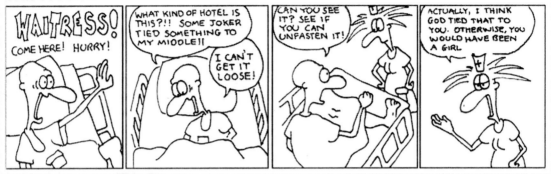
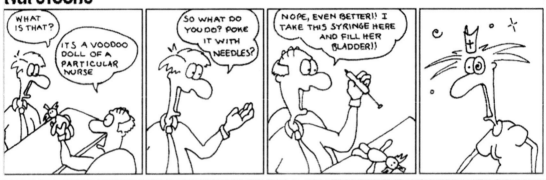
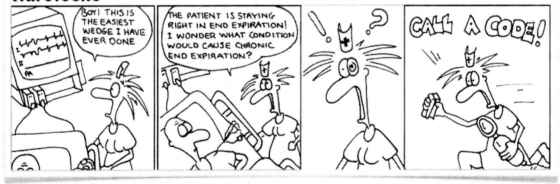

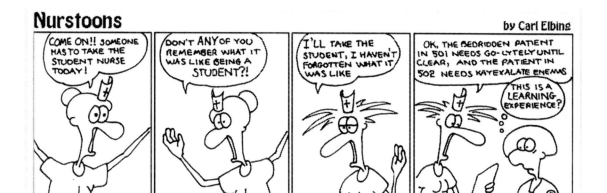
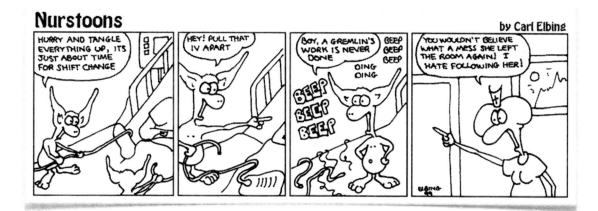
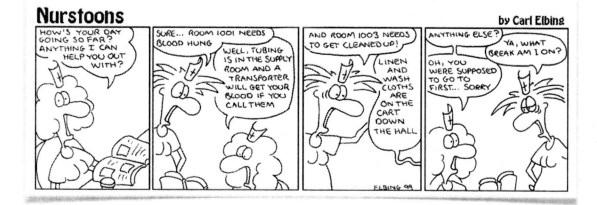

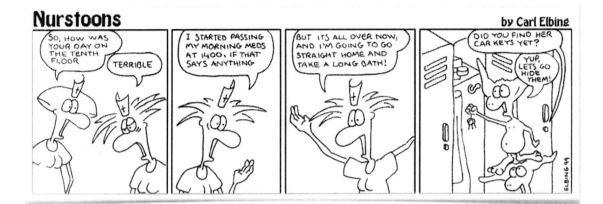
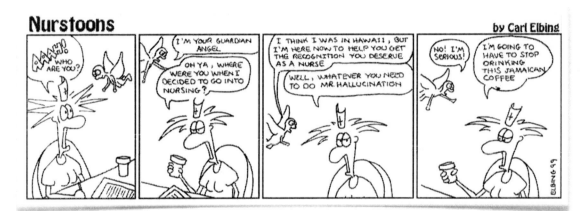
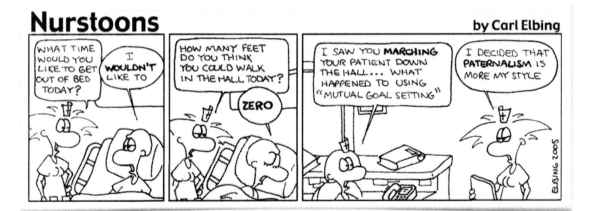

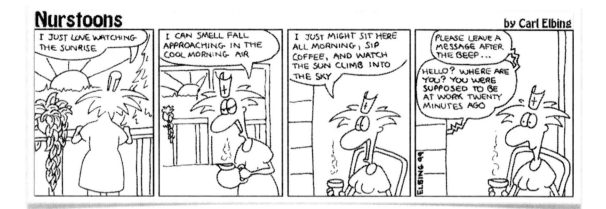
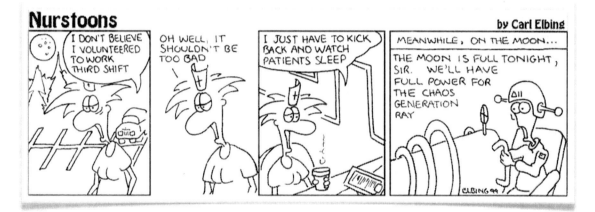
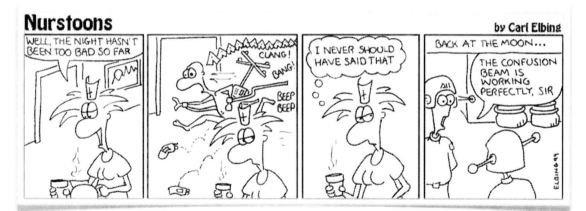

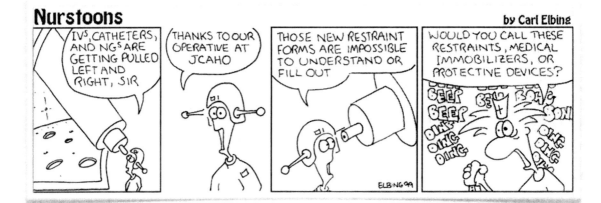
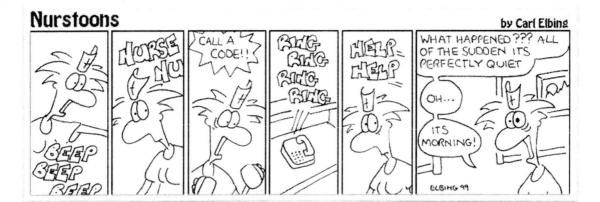
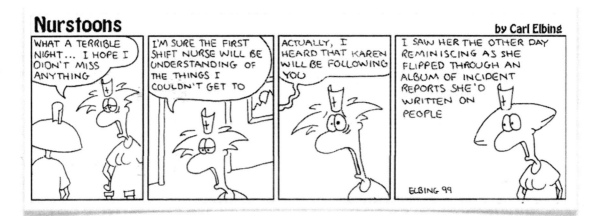

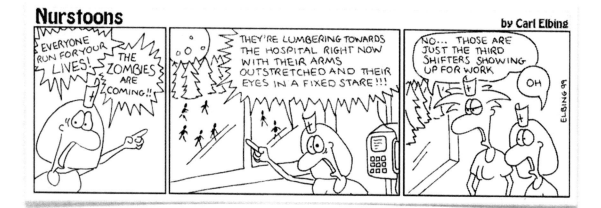
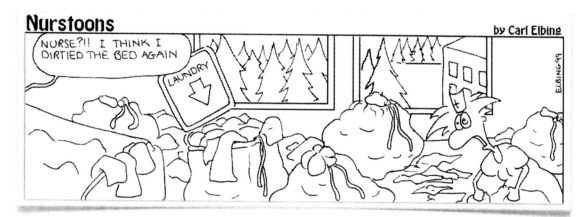
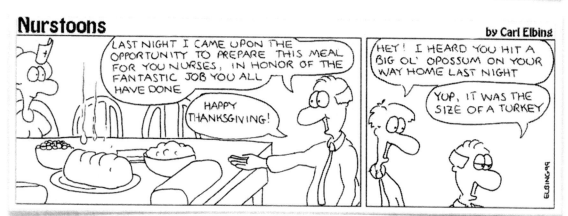

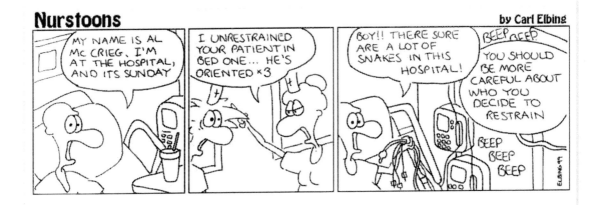
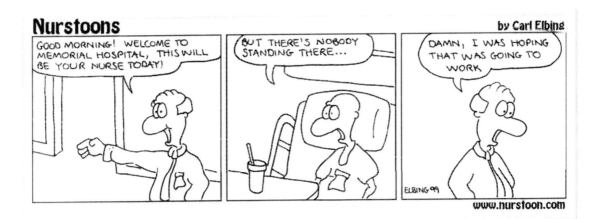
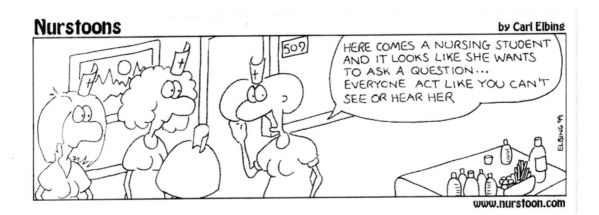

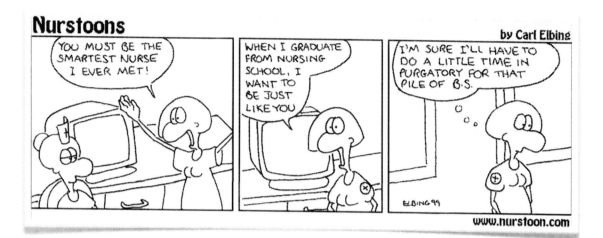
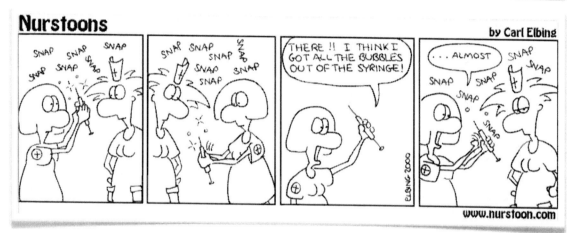
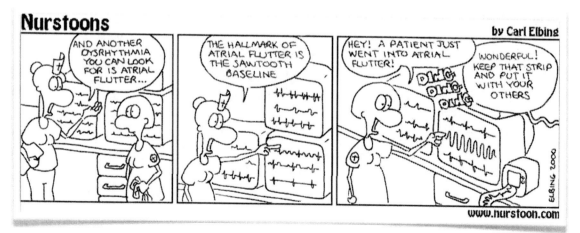

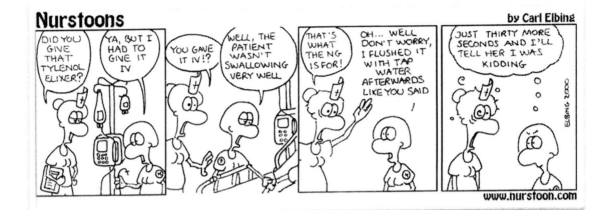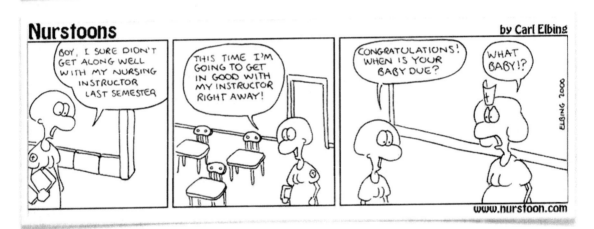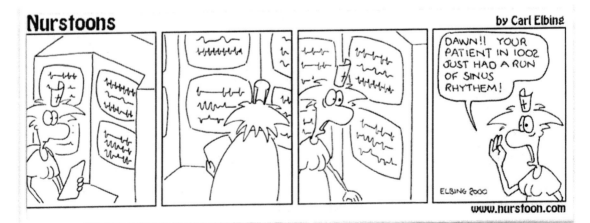

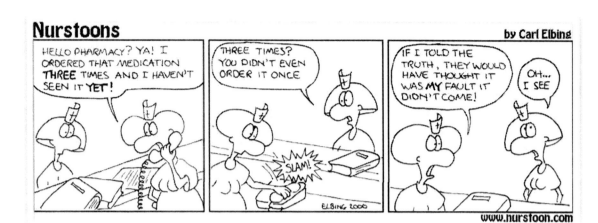
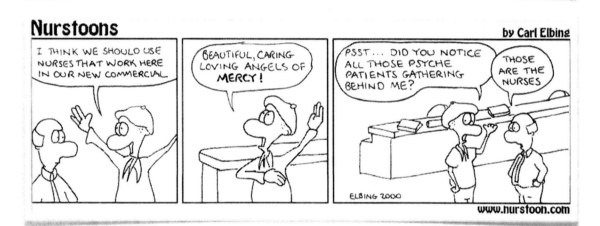
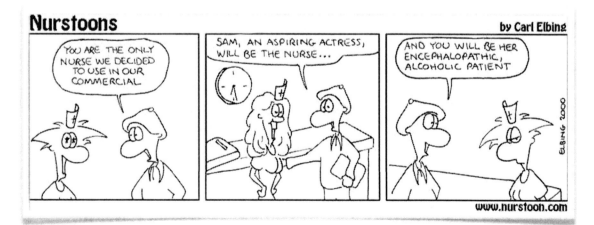

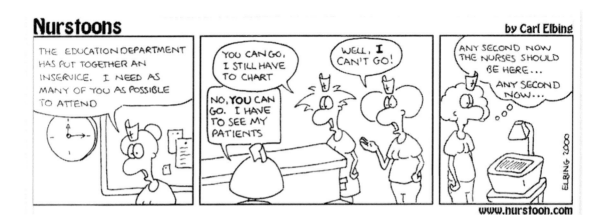
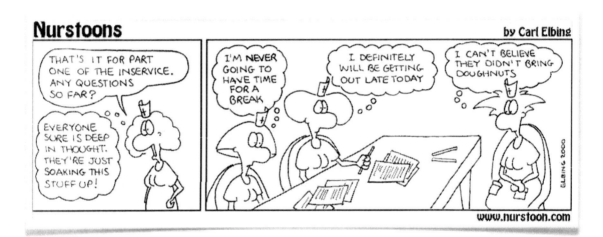
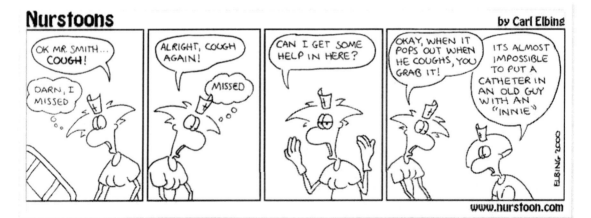

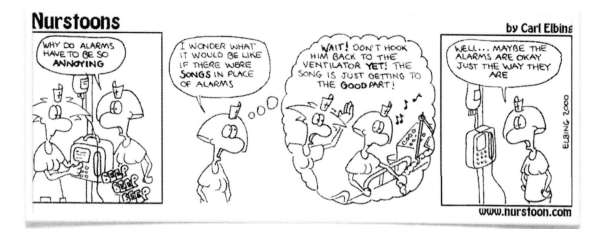
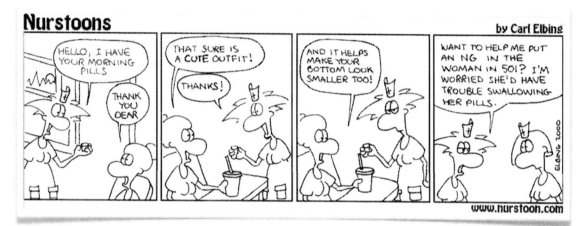
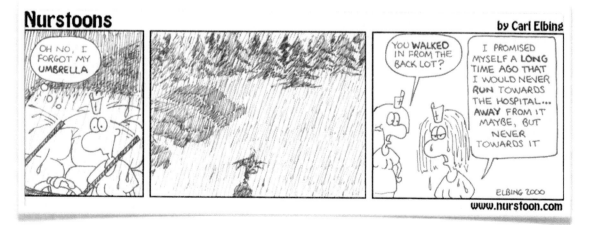

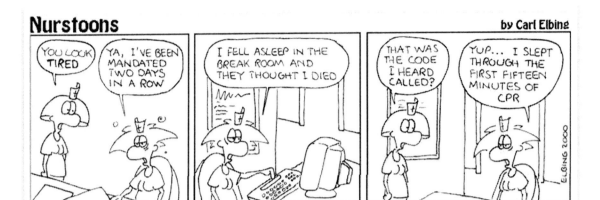

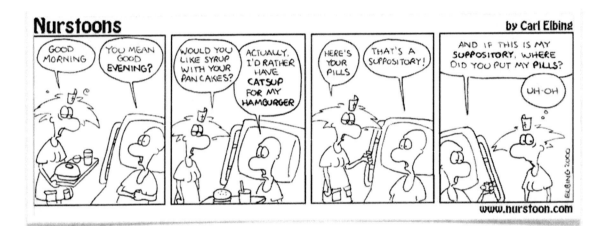

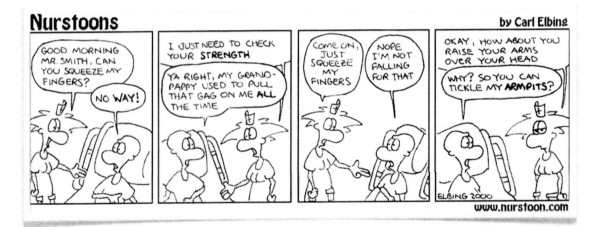

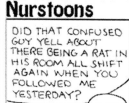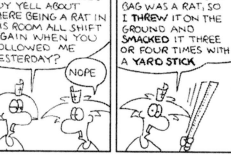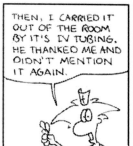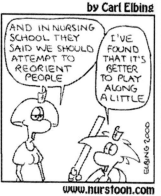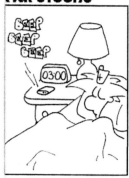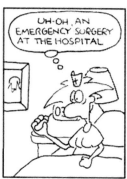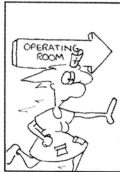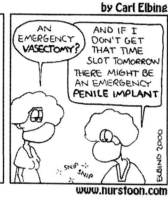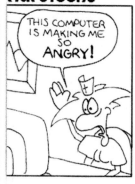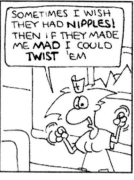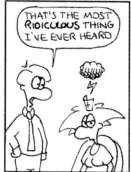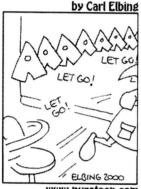

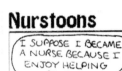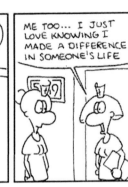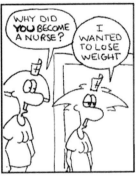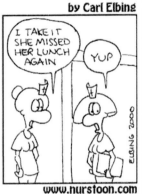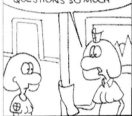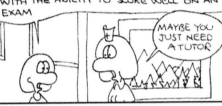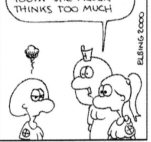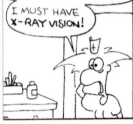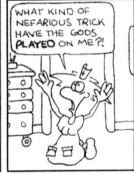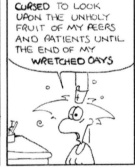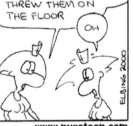

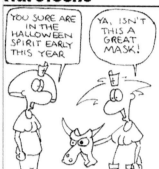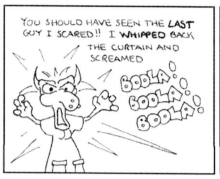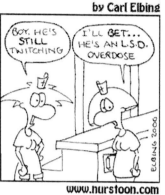
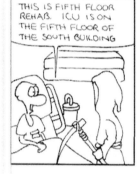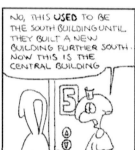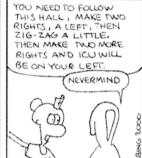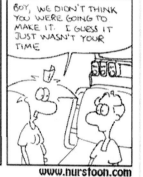
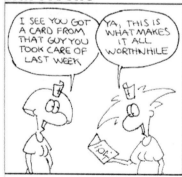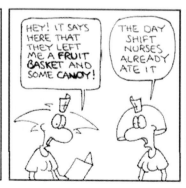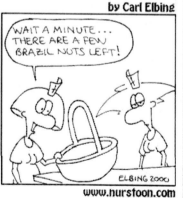

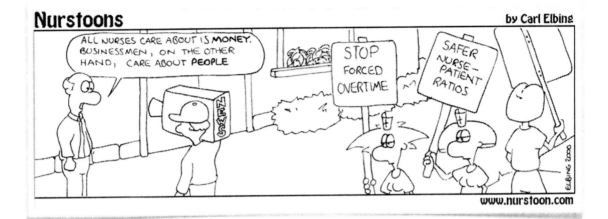
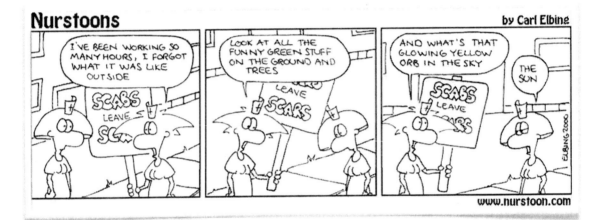
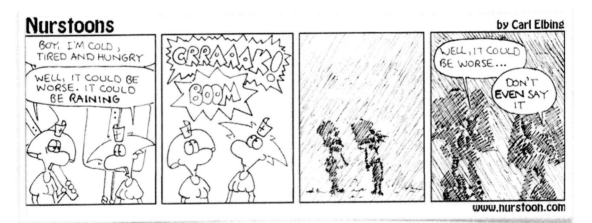

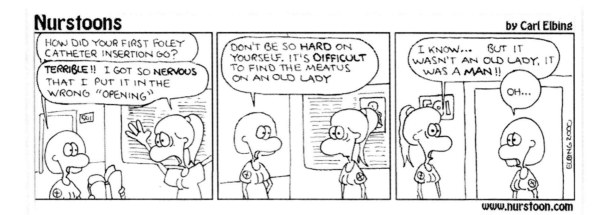
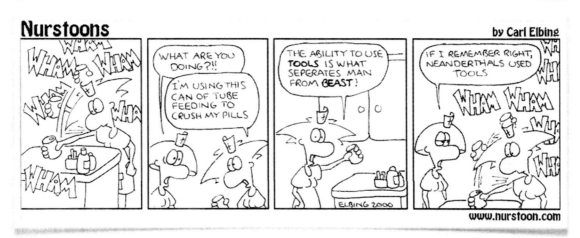
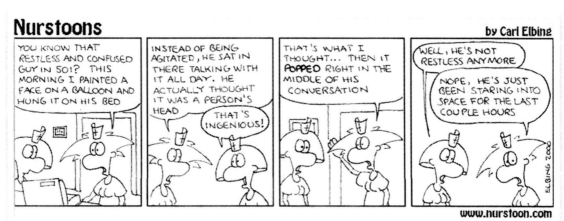

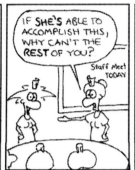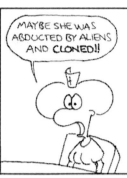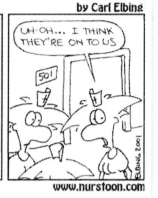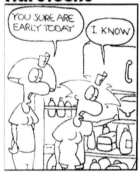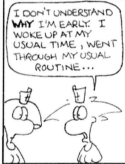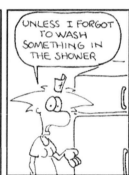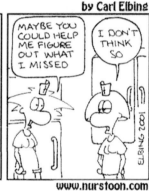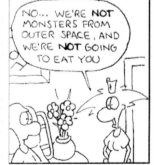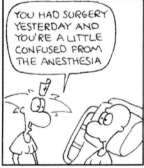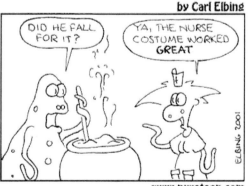

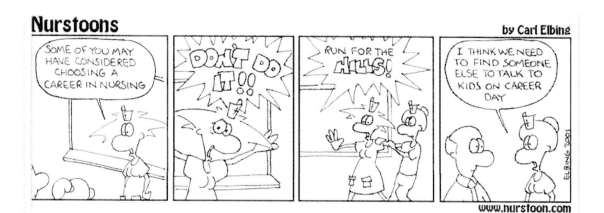
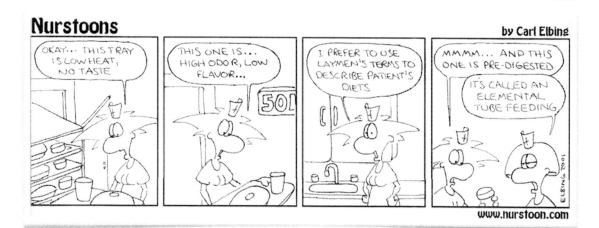
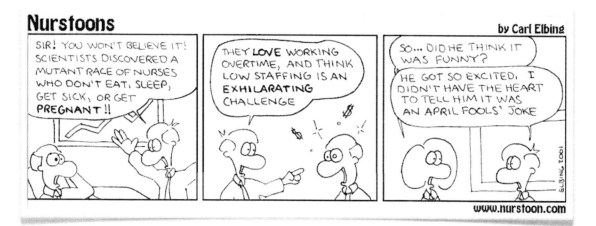

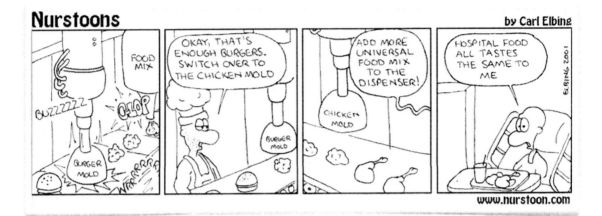
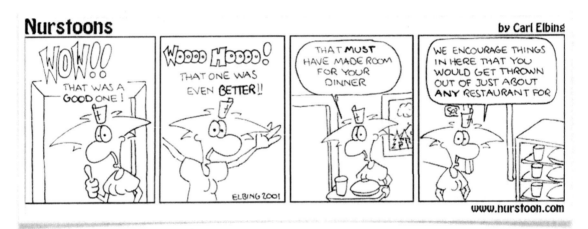
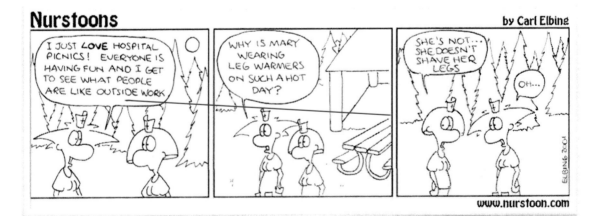

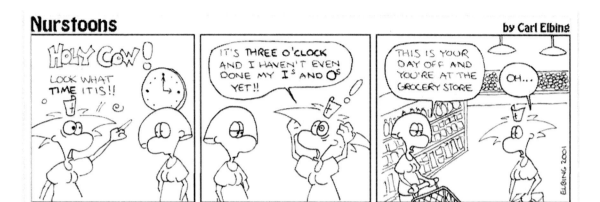
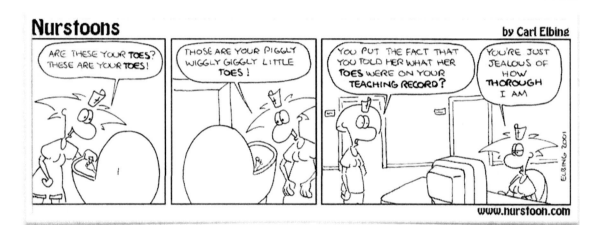
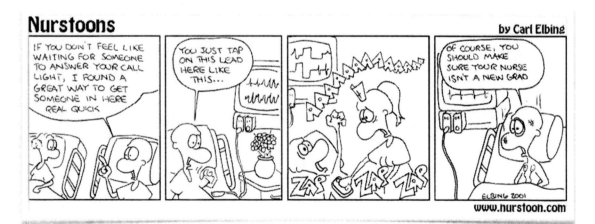

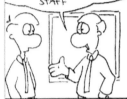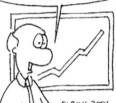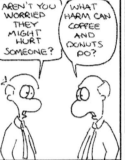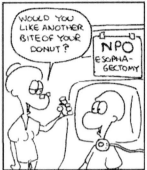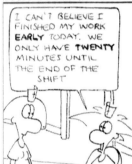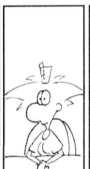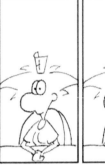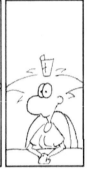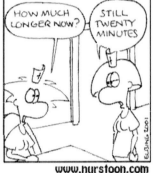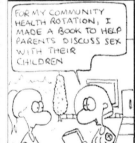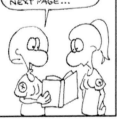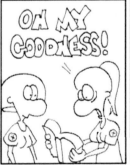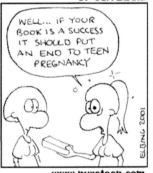

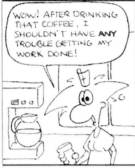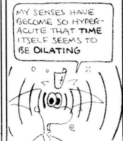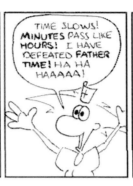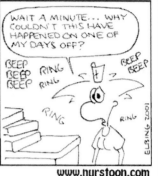
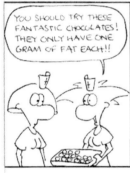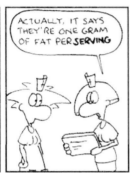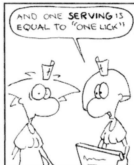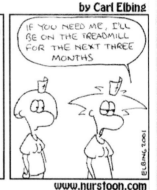
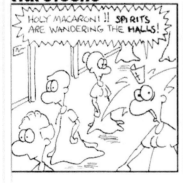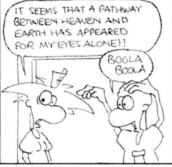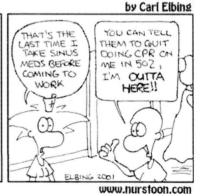

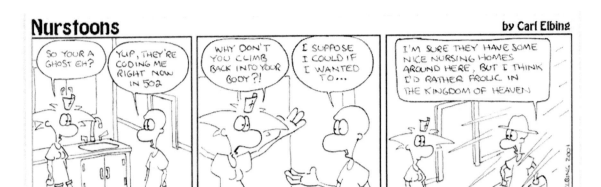
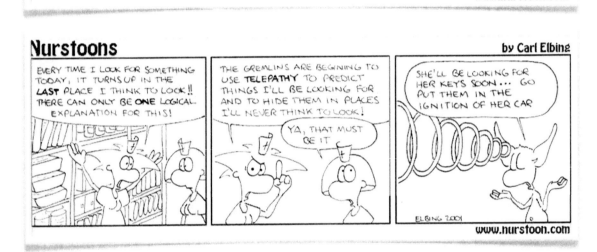
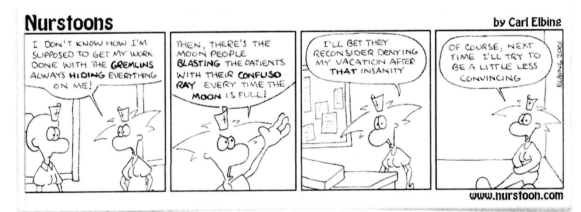

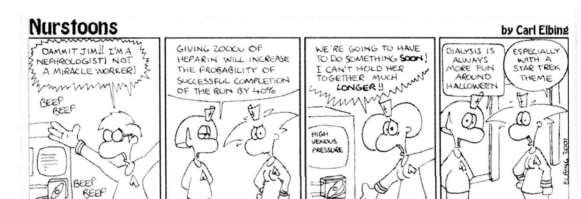
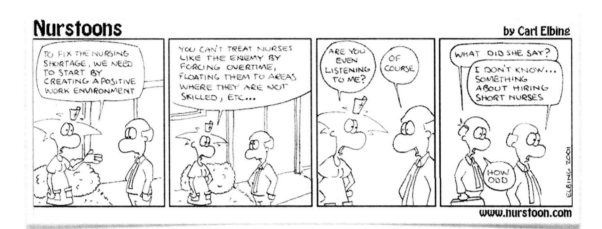
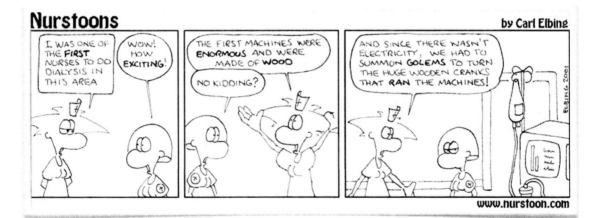

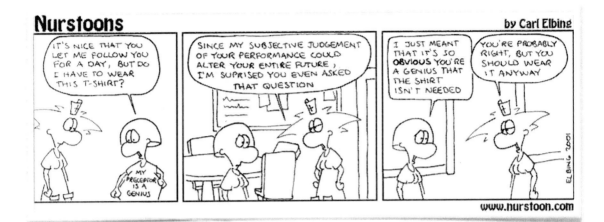
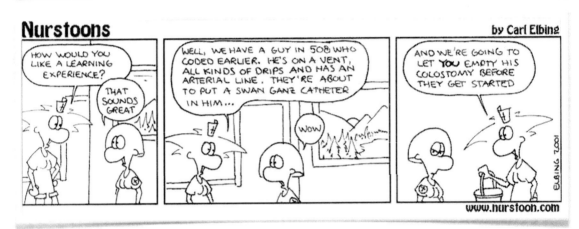
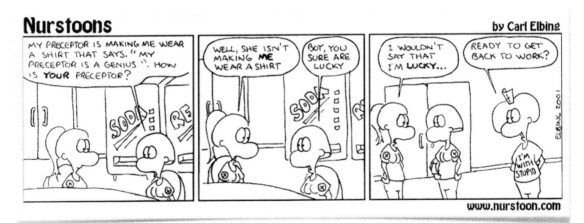

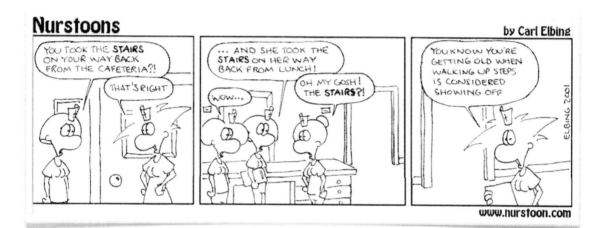
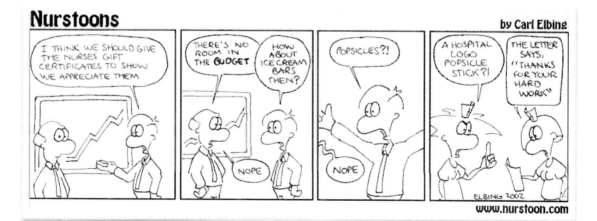

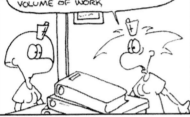
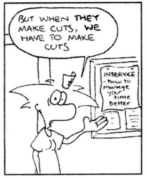
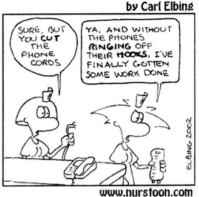
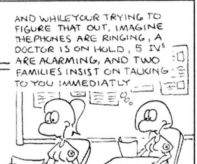
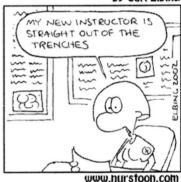
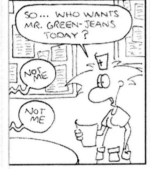
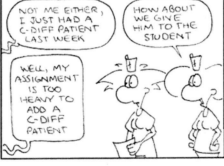

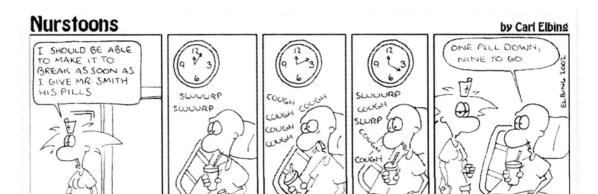
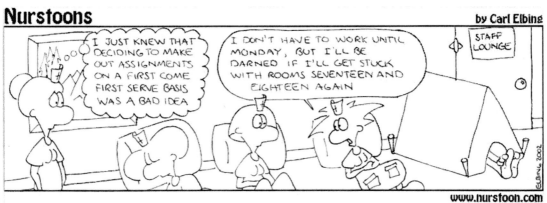
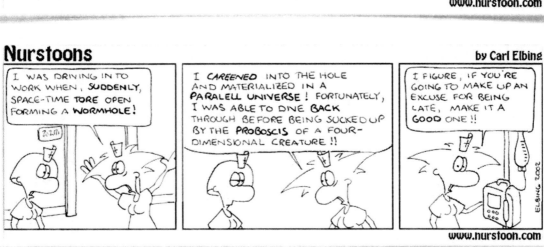

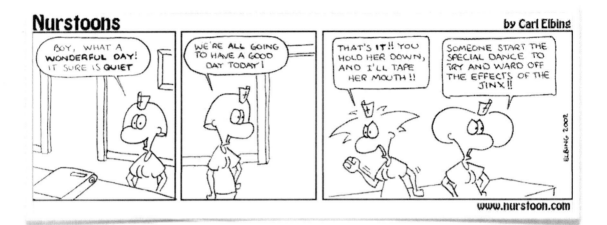
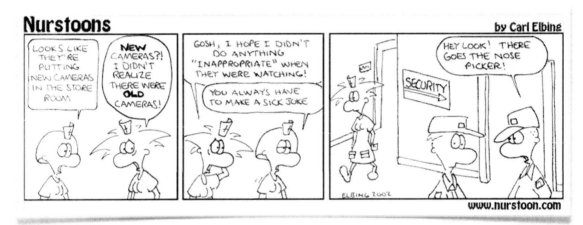
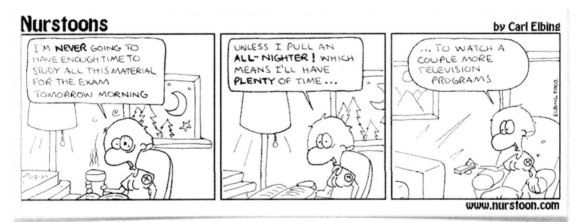

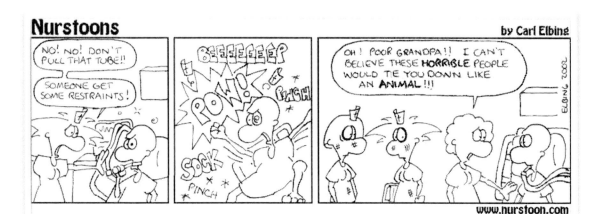
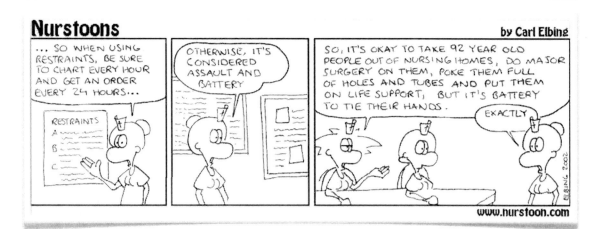
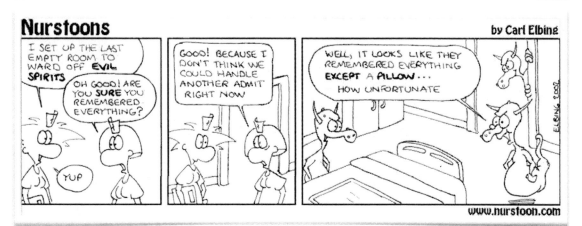

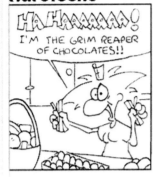
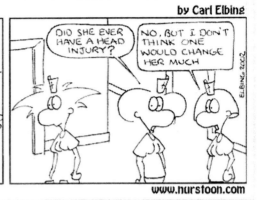
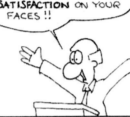
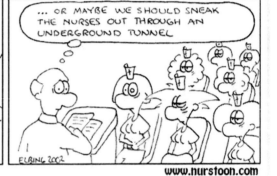
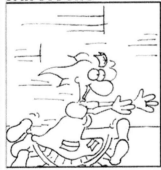
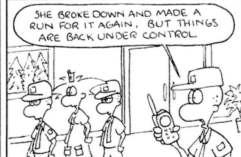

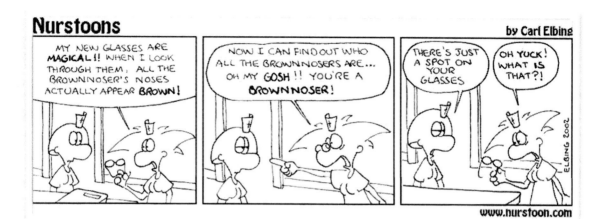
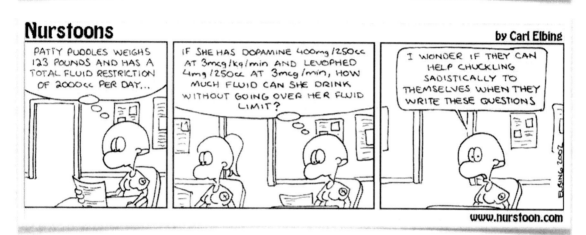
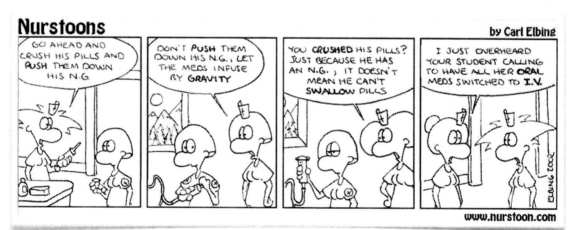

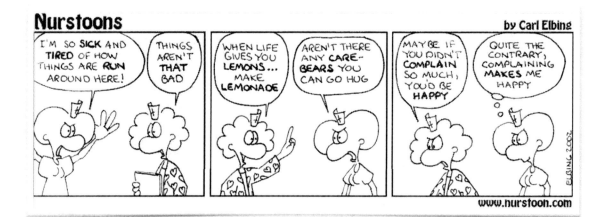
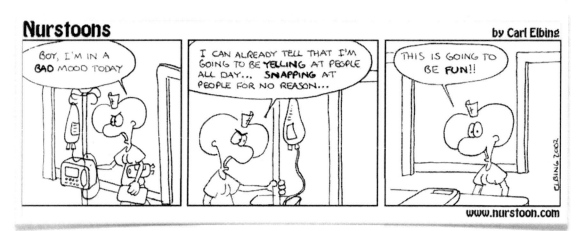
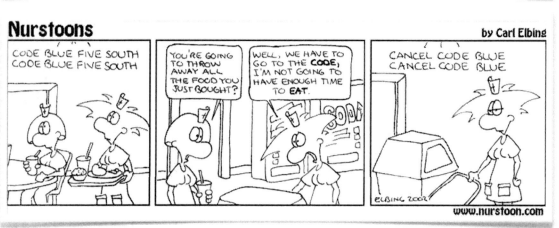

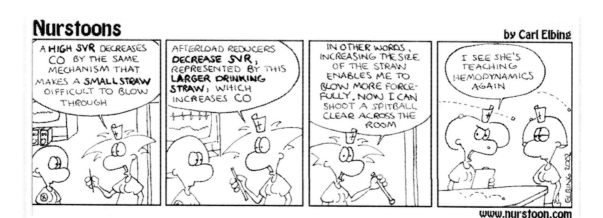
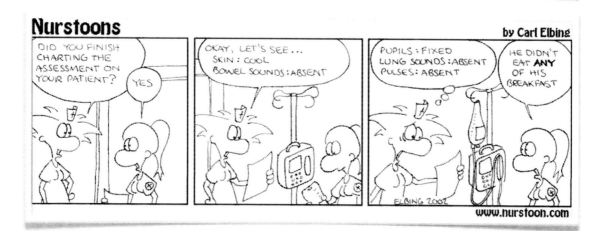
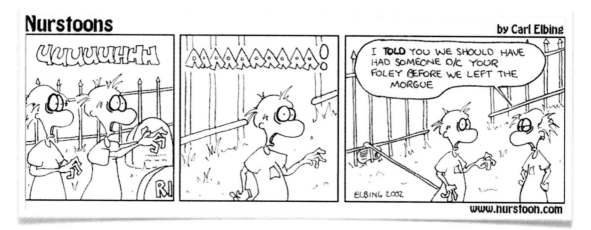

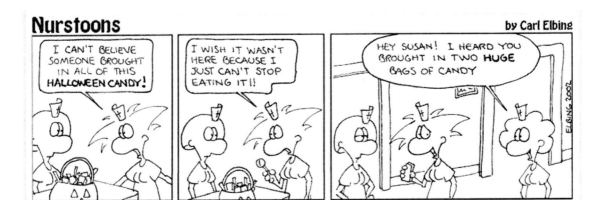
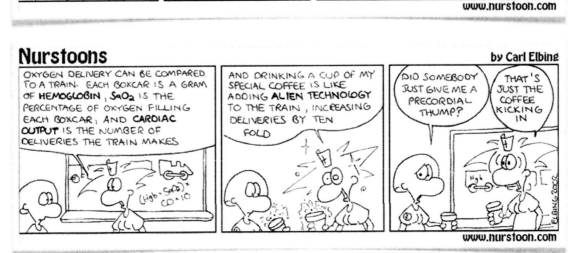
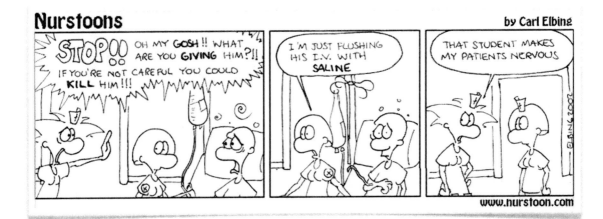

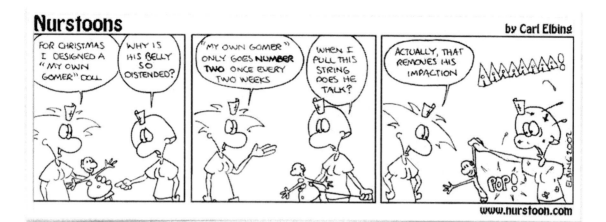
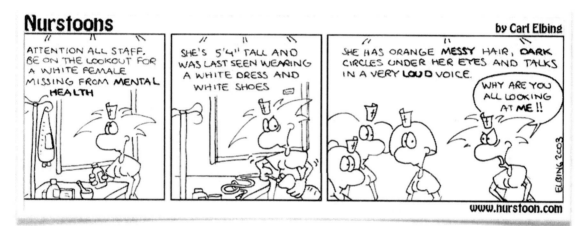
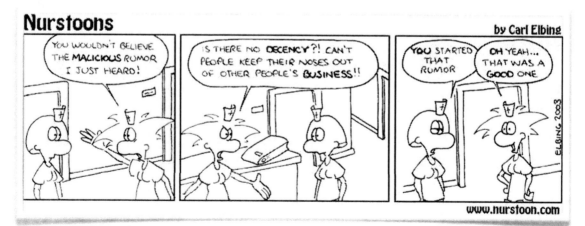

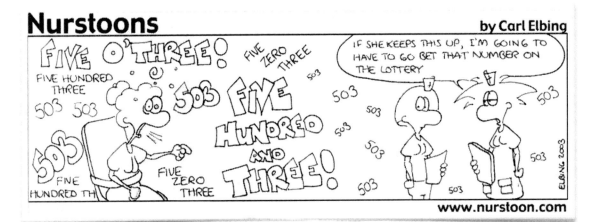
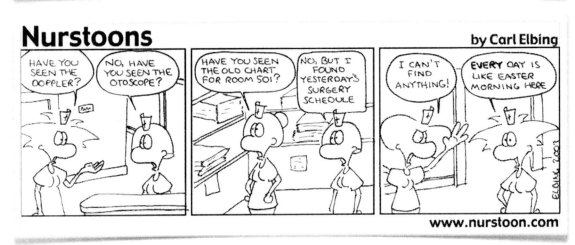
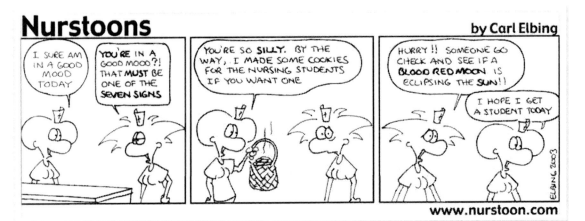

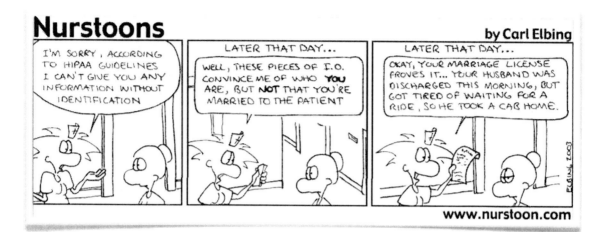
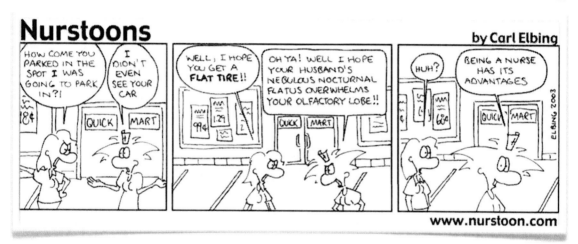
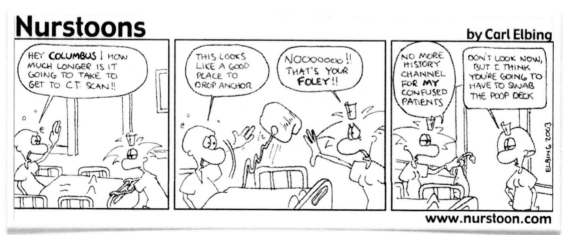

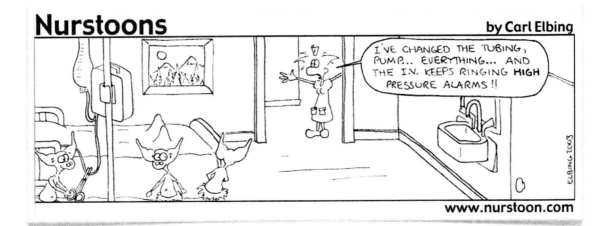
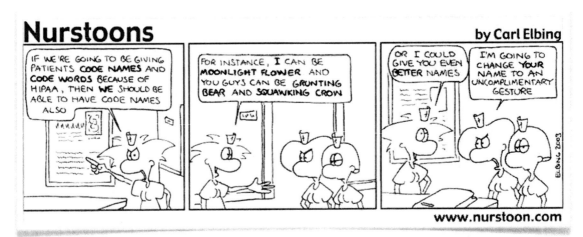
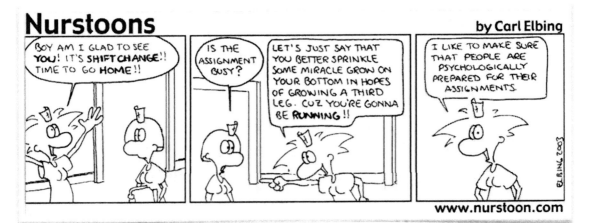

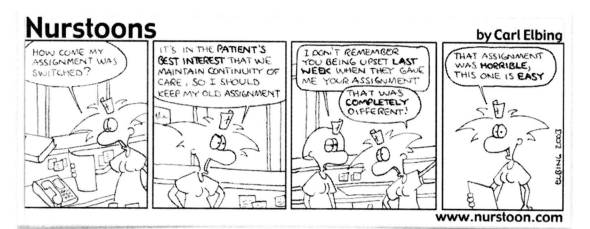
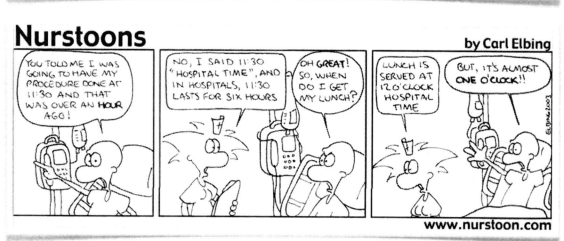
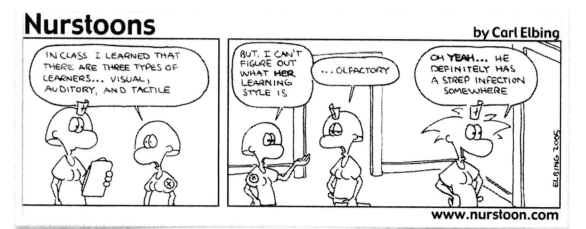

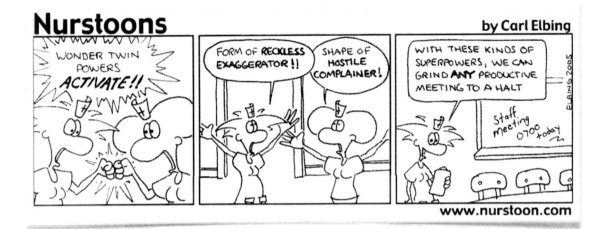
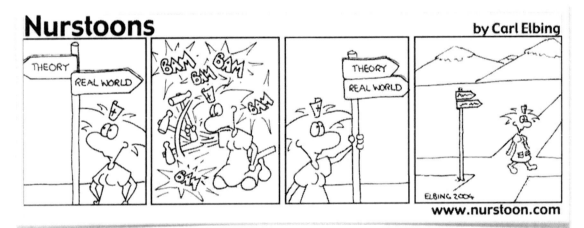
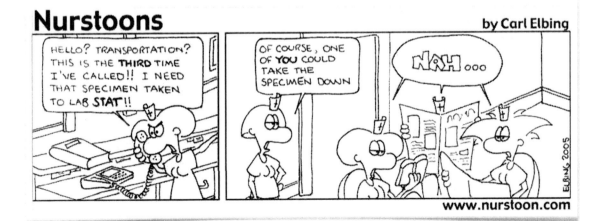

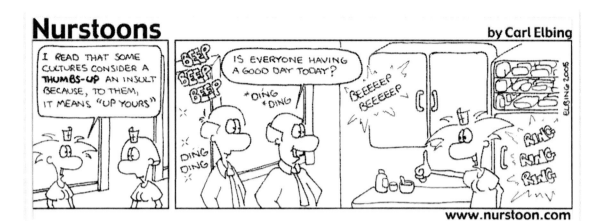
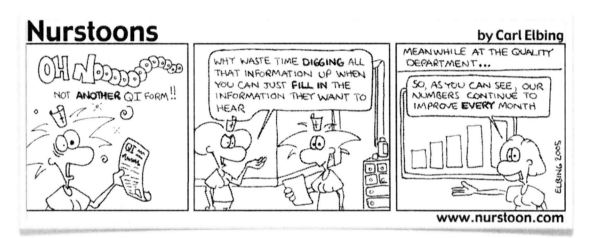
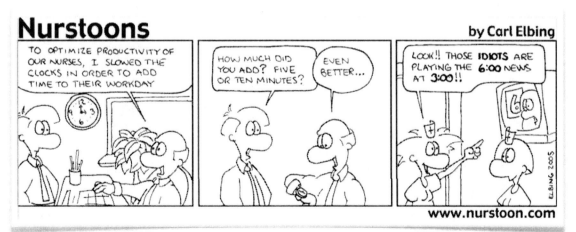

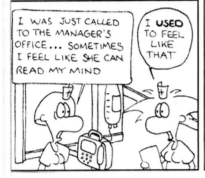
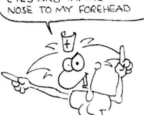
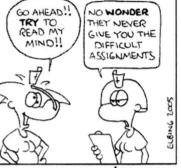
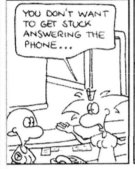
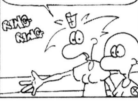
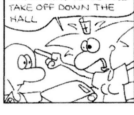
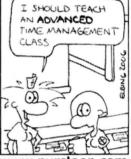
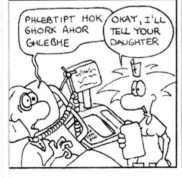
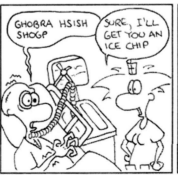
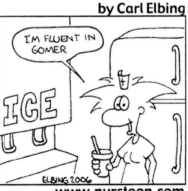

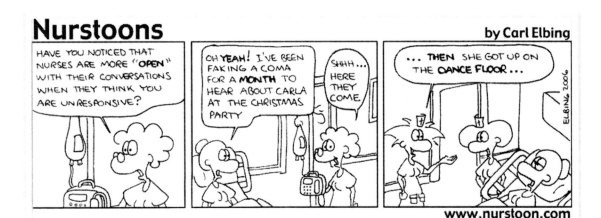
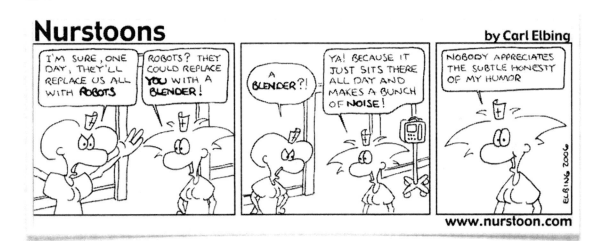
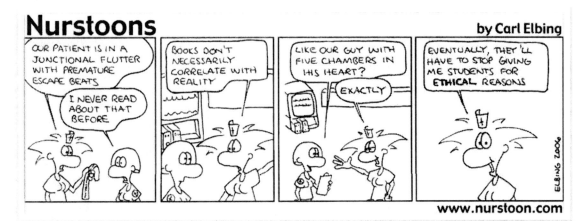

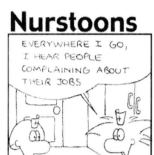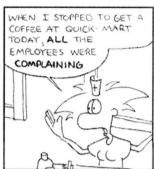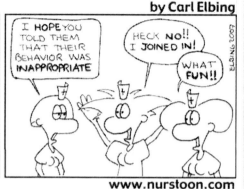
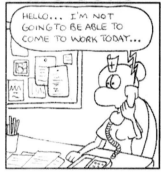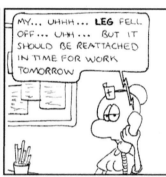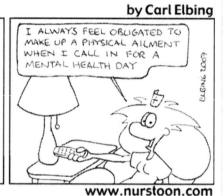
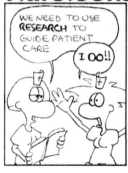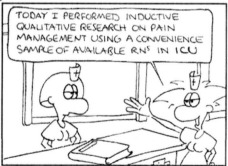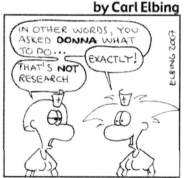

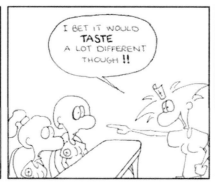
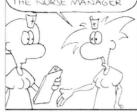
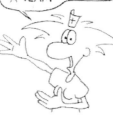
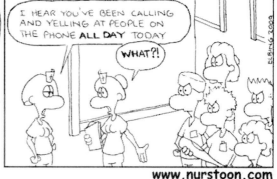
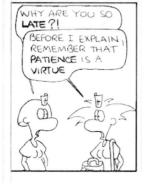
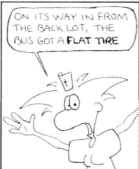

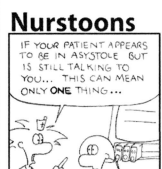
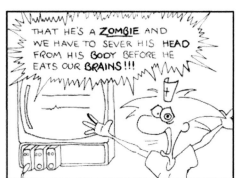
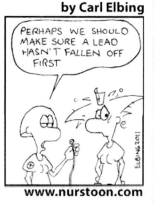
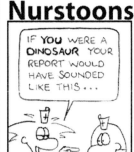
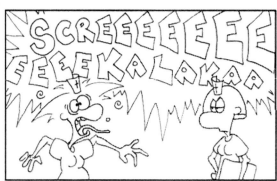
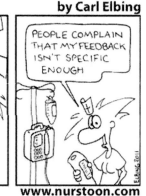
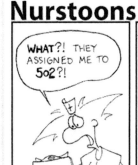
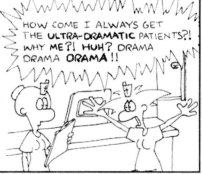
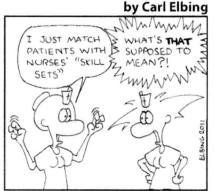

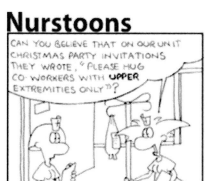
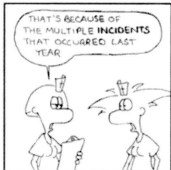
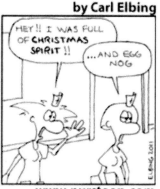
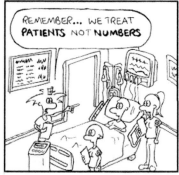
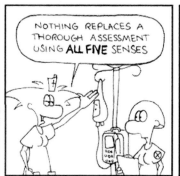
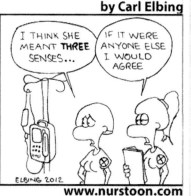
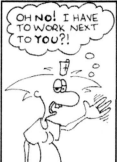
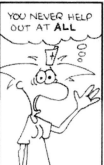
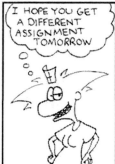
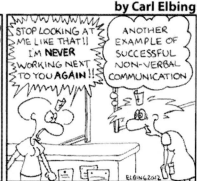

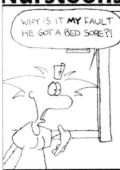
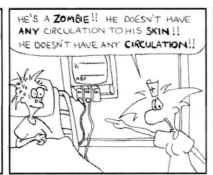
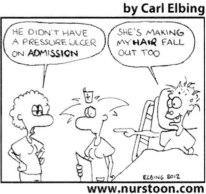
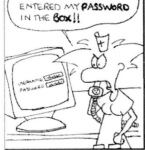
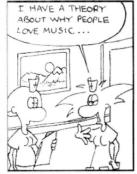
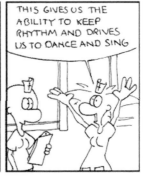

The End

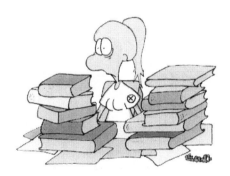

CPSIA information can be obtained at www.ICGtesting.com
Printed in the USA
LVOW110311260413

331065LV00003B/27/P